GERSON THERAPY

Unlocking Healing Potentials, A Comprehensive Guide To Holistic Wellness, Cancer Reversal, Detoxification, Nutrient Restoration, And Disease Prevention

DR. WANDA MENDENHALL

DISCLAIMER

This book is the result of the author's own expertise, insight, and experience in the area of treatment. The author has no affiliation with any particular firm, business, or person mentioned in this article. The content in this book is based exclusively on the author's knowledge and should not be construed as professional advice or a replacement for professional treatment or counseling.

Readers are recommended to seek professional counsel or guidance based on their unique circumstances or requirements. The author and publisher are not liable for any actions done in reliance on the information included in this book. Every person's circumstance is unique, so what works for one person may not work for another.

This book attempts to provide insights and knowledge for both education and personal growth.

The author does not recommend any certain therapy strategy or practice over another. Readers should exercise caution and check with trained specialists before using any knowledge or strategies discussed in this book.

By reading this book, the reader understands and accepts that the author and publisher are not accountable for any direct or indirect repercussions, damages, or losses that occur from the use or misuse of the material included herein.

Table of Contents

INTRODUCTION 12

A Brief Overview Of Gerson Therapy 13

The Historical Evolution Of Gerson Therapy...........15

Purpose And Scope Of The Book.........................16

CHAPTER ONE 20

The Life And Work Of Dr. Max Gerson 20

Early Life And Education 20

Dr. Gerson's Contributions To Medicine 21

Development Of Gerson Therapy Principles..........23

CHAPTER TWO 26

Understanding The Gerson Therapy Protocol 26

Core Principles Of Gerson Therapy 27

   2. Detoxifying: 27

   5. Enzymatic Therapy:.........................28

Dietary Guidelines And Restrictions......................29

   1. .Organic vegetables:..........................29

   2. .Diet:...29

   3. Low Sodium consumption: 30

   4. Elimination of Processed Foods:............30

Importance Of Organic And Fresh Foods...............31

1. Nutritional Density:..31

2. Toxin Avoidance: 31

3. Enzyme Preservation: 32

4. Enhanced Healing capacity:.........................32

CHAPTER THREE 34

The Role Of Juicing In Gerson Therapy...................34

Benefits Of Fresh Juice In Healing 34

4. Enzyme Activation: 36

5. Detoxification: 36

Specific Juicing Protocols.......................................37

2. Variety of Ingredients: 37

Types Of Juices And Their Therapeutic Effects 38

1. Carrot and Apple Juice: 38

3. Cabbage Juice: 39

4. Beet and Liver Support:...............................39

CHAPTER FOUR 42

Detoxification And The Gerson Therapy 42

Liver Detoxification In Gerson Therapy..................43

1. The Liver's Role in Detoxification: 43

2. Plant-Based, Organic, and Nutrient-Rich Diet .43

4. Toxic Load Reduction: 44

Coffee Enemas: Purpose And Procedure 45

1. Introduction to Coffee Enemas: 45

3. Procedure and Frequency: 46

Other Detoxification Methods 46

2. Hydrotherapy: 46

CHAPTER FIVE 50

Nutritional Supplements In Gerson Therapy 50

The Role Of Supplements In Supporting Healing 51

1. Cellular Repair: 51

2. Support for Detoxification: 51

3. Immune System Support:..............................51

4. Critical Organ Support:...............................52

Essential Nutrients And Their Sources 52

1. Vitamins: 52

2. Minerals: 53

3. Enzymes:...53

Balancing The Gerson Diet With Supplements 54

1. Individualized Approaches: 54

2. Monitoring Nutrient Intake:.........................55

3. Avoiding Nutrient Excess: 55

CHAPTER SIX 58

Case Studies And Success Stories 58

Real-Life Experiences Of Gerson Therapy 59

    1. Cases of Cancer Remission: 59

    3. Detoxification and general well-being: 60

Documented Cases Of Healing 60

    1. Scientific Validation: 60

    2. Long-term Follow-ups: 61

Overcoming Challenges In Implementation 61

    1. Compliance with Nutrition: 61

    2. .Juicing and Treatment Routines: 62

    3. .Psychosocial and emotional support: 62

CHAPTER SEVEN 64

Integrating Gerson Therapy With Conventional
Medicine 64

Gerson Therapy And Its Relationship With
Conventional Treatments 64

    1. .Nutritional Focus: 65

    2. .Detoxification and mainstream Treatments: 65

Collaborative Approaches To Healing 67

    2. .Patient-Centered Care: 67

    3. .Protocol Monitoring and Adjustment: 68

Addressing Criticisms And Concerns 69

1. .Scientific Evidence and Research:.................69

2. .Communication and Transparency: 69

3. .Patient Education:....................................70

CHAPTER EIGHT..72

Gerson Therapy And Chronic Illnesses 72

Gerson Therapy In Cancer Treatment 72

4. .Immune System Support:...........................74

Application In Other Chronic Conditions...............74

1. .Autoimmune Diseases: 75

2. .Cardiovascular Diseases: 75

3. .Digestive issues:.......................................76

Managing Chronic Diseases With A Holistic
Approach...76

1. Nutritional Healing:...................................77

2. Detoxification: 77

4. Individualized therapy: 78

CHAPTER NINE 80

Practical Tips For Implementing Gerson Therapy ...80

Creating A Gerson-Friendly Environment At Home 81

1. .Availability of Organic Produce: 81

2. .Juicing Station:..............................81

4. .Water Filtration:..............................82

5. .Natural Cleaning Products:.....................82

Meal Planning And Preparation........................83

1. .Weekly Meal Plans:............................83

2. .Batch cooking:................................83

3. .Preparation of items:.........................84

4. .Variety and Creativity:.......................84

Overcoming Common Obstacles..........................84

1. .Social Difficulties:.........................84

2. .Time Management:..............................85

3. .Financial Considerations:.....................85

CHAPTER TEN..88

The Future Of Gerson Therapy.........................88

Ongoing Research And Developments....................89

2. .Nutritional Optimization:.....................89

Potential Advancements In Gerson-Inspired Protocols...90

1. .Integration with Modern Medicine:.............90

2. .Detoxification Protocol Innovations:..........91

3. .Technological Integration:....................91

Promoting Awareness And Accessibility 92

    1. .Education Initiatives: 92

    2. .Patient Support Networks: 92

    3. .Training Treatment Professionals: 93

    4. .Research financing: 93

Conclusion 95

THE END 99

INTRODUCTION

Gerson Therapy is a comprehensive alternative therapy technique created by Dr. Max Gerson in the early twentieth century that focuses on employing a specific diet, detoxification, and nutritional supplements to address and prevent different chronic illnesses, with a special emphasis on cancer.

This treatment regimen is based on the notion that, given the correct tools and circumstances, the body has a natural potential to repair itself. This review of Gerson Therapy delves into its historical growth, the principles underlying its application, as well as the goal and scope of this therapeutic technique.

A Brief Overview Of Gerson Therapy

Gerson Therapy is an all-inclusive, integrative therapy plan that incorporates dietary modifications, cleansing procedures, and nutritional supplements to activate the body's inherent healing processes.

An organic, plant-based diet, regular fresh juices, coffee enemas, and avoidance of particular toxins are key components of the treatment. Gerson Therapy's nutritional component stresses the eating of fresh, organic fruits and vegetables while avoiding processed meals, meat, dairy, and refined carbohydrates.

Gerson Therapy is based on the idea that an alkaline, plant-based diet high in nutrients and enzymes might help the body cleanse and repair damaged cells. The treatment tries to rebalance the body, boost the immune system, and create an environment in which cancer cells cannot survive.

It is used to treat a variety of chronic ailments, including autoimmune diseases and degenerative disorders, in addition to cancer.

Gerson Therapy has its origins in the early twentieth century, when Dr. Max Gerson, a German-born physician, started developing his holistic approach to healing. Dr. Gerson's research began with him treating his migraines, and through diet and nutrition testing, he discovered the significant influence that specific foods might have on health. As his studies progressed, he found excellent results in individuals suffering from a variety of chronic conditions, including TB and cancer.

Dr. Gerson escaped Nazi Germany in the 1930s and finally resided in the United

States. He proceeded to refine and promote his therapeutic technique, receiving prominence for its supposed efficacy in cancer treatment. Gerson Therapy gained popularity despite objections from certain mainstream medical circles, and Dr. Gerson published his results in the book "A Cancer Therapy: Results of Fifty Cases."

Purpose And Scope Of The Book

The goal of this book is to give a thorough examination of Gerson Therapy, including its principles, historical history, and use in the treatment of chronic disorders, including cancer. Readers will acquire insights into the holistic concepts that underlie this alternative approach to health and well-being by investigating the underlying philosophy and technique of Gerson Therapy.

The book's breadth goes beyond just detailing the therapy's history and ideas. It seeks to give a fair viewpoint, delving into both the claims of proponents and the critiques and issues surrounding Gerson Therapy. Furthermore, the book will cover the present state of Gerson Therapy in the context of modern healthcare, addressing its integration with conventional medicine and its role in the spectrum of available therapeutic alternatives.

In short, this book tries to present readers with a comprehensive knowledge of Gerson Therapy, providing insights into its historical background, the opinions of its proponents, and its prospective influence on the landscape of alternative and integrative medicine.

CHAPTER ONE

The Life And Work Of Dr. Max Gerson

Early Life And Education

Dr. Max Gerson was born in Wongrowitz, a tiny village in Germany, on October 18. 1881. . His childhood was defined by a strong interest in science and medicine.

Gerson started his schooling at the University of Würzburg, where he studied medicine. Later, he proceeded to the University of Freiburg, where he graduated with honors in 1909. . Gerson's medical school years laid the groundwork for his future contributions to alternative medicine.

Dr. Gerson's Contributions To Medicine

Dr. Gerson's medical career was marked by a search for novel and holistic ways of treatment. He was a research fellow at the renowned Albert Schweitzer Institute in Frankfurt in the early twentieth century, focused on experimental pathology. Gerson's early study set the framework for his subsequent nutrition and detoxification ideas.

Dr. Gerson's study on migraines was one of his most important achievements. He published publications in the 1920s on the relationship between nutrition and migraine episodes, implying that dietary adjustments might ameliorate symptoms. This paper exemplified his early concern with the influence of diet on health, a concept that would later become important to Gerson's therapeutic approach.

Dr. Gerson's study grew throughout time to include a broad spectrum of chronic and degenerative disorders. To address these illnesses, he investigated the impact of food, detoxification, and the body's inherent healing capabilities. Gerson's holistic approach contrasted with traditional medicine at the time, stressing the interdependence of many physiological systems and the significance of treating the underlying causes of disorders.

Development Of Gerson Therapy Principles

Dr. Gerson proceeded to deepen his knowledge of the link between nutrition and health throughout the 1920s and 1930s, laying the groundwork for Gerson Therapy. His observations and studies resulted in the development of a complete food and detoxification plan intended to promote the body's natural capacity to repair itself.

Gerson Therapy's key concepts are the eating of fresh, organic fruits and vegetables, especially juices, and the avoidance of processed and refined meals. Coffee enemas, which Dr. Gerson thought were important in increasing liver cleansing, are also included in the treatment.

Dr. Max Gerson's foundational publication, "A Cancer Therapy: Results of Fifty Cases," was published in 1958. explaining the concepts and results of Gerson Therapy in the treatment of cancer. The book included case studies that showed exceptional improvements and remissions in individuals who followed the Gerson Protocol.

Gerson Therapy gained popularity because of its holistic and natural approach to healing, but it was also criticized by the medical establishment. Despite obstacles, Dr. Gerson's legacy lives on as many people and practitioners continue to investigate and advocate for Gerson Therapy concepts in the search for alternative and complementary methods of health and healing.

CHAPTER TWO

Understanding The Gerson Therapy Protocol

Gerson Therapy is a comprehensive and intense dietary strategy created by Dr. Max Gerson in the 1920s to treat and prevent numerous chronic illnesses, with a major emphasis on cancer.

This chapter digs into the essential concepts of Gerson Therapy, explaining the protocol's dietary rules and limits and highlighting the critical relevance of organic and fresh foods.

1. .Gerson Therapy promotes the eating of nutrient-dense meals, particularly plant-based foods, to give the body vital vitamins, minerals, enzymes, and other bioactive components. The protocol's goal is to strengthen the immune system and aid the body's natural healing processes.

2. **Detoxifying:** The treatment emphasizes detoxifying via greater consumption of fresh fruits and vegetables. The liver, a vital organ in detoxification, is aided by the ingestion of nutrients that improve its function.

3. Gerson Therapy advocates for an alkaline environment in the body,

claiming that illnesses flourish in an acidic environment. The foods advised are largely alkaline-forming, which helps to maintain an ideal pH balance.

4. Fresh, raw fruit and vegetable juices are consumed on a regular basis as part of the treatment. These juices provide concentrated nutrients in an easily digested form, so assisting the body's healing systems.

5. **Enzymatic Therapy:** It is claimed that including raw and enzyme-rich meals helps to boost the enzymatic processes required for digestion and general health. Raw fruits and vegetables include natural enzymes that help in nutritional absorption.

1. **.Organic vegetables:** Gerson Therapy strongly advises avoiding pesticides, herbicides, and other chemicals by eating organic vegetables. According to the regimen, organic foods are higher in nutrients and devoid of dangerous elements that might impede the healing process.

2. **.Diet:** The treatment advocates for a largely vegetarian and plant-based diet, with a concentration on fresh fruits and vegetables. This diet is thought to provide critical nutrients to the body while limiting the consumption of potentially

hazardous chemicals present in animal products.

3. Low Sodium consumption: Gerson Therapy limits sodium consumption since too much salt is thought to contribute to illness development. The guideline discourages the use of table salt and promotes the eating of naturally low-sodium foods.

4. Elimination of Processed Foods: Gerson Therapy discourages the use of processed foods, which often include additives, preservatives, and other synthetic components. To enhance nutritional advantages, the emphasis is on complete, unprocessed foods.

Importance Of Organic And Fresh Foods

1.   **Nutritional Density:** Organic and fresh foods are thought to have more nutritional content than conventionally produced and processed alternatives. These nutrient-dense meals are used in Gerson Therapy to give the body with the necessary building blocks for recovery.

2. **Toxin Avoidance:** Eating organic foods reduces your chances of being exposed to pesticides, herbicides, and other agricultural chemicals. To promote the body's detoxification processes, the treatment stresses the necessity of reducing the toxic burden.

3. Enzyme Preservation: Fresh foods, particularly fresh fruits and vegetables, preserve their natural enzymes, which are thought to play an important role in digestion and nutritional absorption. Gerson Therapy tries to optimize health by harnessing these enzymes.

4. Enhanced Healing capacity: It is believed that the lack of toxins in organic and fresh meals enhances the body's healing capacity. According to Gerson Therapy, a clean, nutrient-rich diet helps to a more conducive environment for healing.

Finally, Chapter Two of Gerson Therapy thoroughly examines the protocol's key concepts, specifies dietary requirements and limits, and emphasizes the critical need to select organic and fresh foods to assist healing and improve general well-being.

CHAPTER THREE

The Role Of Juicing In Gerson Therapy

Juicing is essential in Dr. Max Gerson's Gerson Therapy, a comprehensive approach to curing and treating chronic illnesses. This chapter delves into the advantages of fresh juice in the healing process, particular juicing procedures, and the therapeutic effects of different kinds of juices.

Benefits Of Fresh Juice In Healing

1. .Freshly squeezed juices made from organic fruits and vegetables are high in vitamins, minerals, enzymes, and phytonutrients. These nutrients are critical

for strengthening the immune system and supporting the body's natural healing processes.

2. Juicing aids in the maintenance of adequate cellular hydration by supplying the body with a concentrated dose of water as well as critical nutrients. Hydration is essential for general health and assists in the removal of toxins from the body.

3. Many illnesses flourish in an acidic environment, therefore the alkalizing effect is beneficial. Gerson Therapy promotes the intake of alkaline-forming foods, and freshly juiced fruits and vegetables help to create a more alkaline

internal environment, which is thought to slow disease development.

4. Enzyme Activation: Enzymes found in raw fruits and vegetables aid digestion and nutritional absorption. Juicing maintains these enzymes, assisting in the digestion of the juice's nutrients and lowering the load on the digestive system.

5. Detoxification: Gerson Therapy focuses on detoxifying the body to remove poisons that have accumulated. The nutrients in fresh juices aid in the detoxification processes of the liver, boosting the elimination of toxic chemicals from the body.

1. Gerson Therapy suggests drinking fresh juices often throughout the day. Patients often drink several glasses of juice between meals to guarantee a steady supply of nutrients.

2. **Variety of Ingredients:** The treatment encourages for the juices to include a wide variety of fruits and vegetables. This diversity guarantees a diverse range of nutrients while also enhancing the medicinal benefits of the juices.

3. Juices are often drunk separately from meals in order to maximize vitamin absorption. Patients are recommended to take their juices at least 30 minutes before

and after meals, enabling the body to concentrate on digestion throughout mealtime.

Types Of Juices And Their Therapeutic Effects

1. Carrot and Apple Juice: A staple of Gerson Therapy, carrot and apple juice is strong in beta-carotene and contains critical elements for healing. It has anti-inflammatory and immune-boosting effects.

2. Green juices are high in chlorophyll and antioxidants and are frequently produced from a blend of leafy greens such as kale, spinach, and celery. These juices aid in cleansing and oxygenation of

the body, as well as general cellular health.

3. Cabbage Juice: Cabbage juice is used to treat gastrointestinal ailments due to its anti-inflammatory and healing characteristics. It is said to help with illnesses including ulcers and gastritis.

4. Beet and Liver Support: Beet juice, typically coupled with additional nutrients, is recognized for enhancing blood health and supporting liver function. It is an important part of Gerson Therapy for detoxification.

In conclusion, juicing has a diverse function in Gerson Therapy, including nutritional replacement, hydration, detoxification, and immunological support. The precise protocols and juice types indicated in the treatment are adapted to the specific requirements of people undergoing the healing process. As a key component of Gerson Therapy, freshly squeezed juices contribute greatly to the holistic approach to health and fitness.

CHAPTER FOUR

Detoxification And The Gerson Therapy

Detoxification is an essential component in Dr. Max Gerson's Gerson Therapy, a holistic and alternative method to treating chronic illnesses.

This chapter delves into the relevance of detoxification in Gerson Therapy, with a particular emphasis on liver detoxification, the use of coffee enemas, and other detoxification procedures used in this therapeutic approach.

1. The Liver's Role in Detoxification: The liver is essential in detoxification because it processes and eliminates toxins from the body. Improving liver function is an important part of the Gerson Therapy procedure.

2. Plant-Based, Organic, and Nutrient-Rich Diet: Gerson Therapy stresses a plant-based, organic, and nutrient-dense diet. The treatment helps the liver's natural detoxification processes by giving the body with necessary vitamins and minerals.

3.   .Freshly squeezed organic fruit and vegetable juices, a cornerstone of Gerson Therapy, are thought to give the body enzymes that aid in cleansing. These juices are ingested throughout the day to aid cellular regeneration and to improve the liver's capacity to remove toxins.

4. **Toxic Load Reduction:** Gerson Therapy advocates for limiting the consumption of processed foods, chemicals, and environmental contaminants. This decrease in toxic load on the body is supposed to lighten the pressure on the liver and speed up the detoxification process.

1. Introduction to Coffee Enemas: The use of coffee enemas as a detoxifying therapy is a distinguishing aspect of the Gerson Therapy. Coffee enemas include the rectal injection of coffee solution and are thought to stimulate the liver and improve toxin removal.

2. Coffee is considered to boost bile production in the liver because it contains chemicals that stimulate bile formation. Increased bile flow is thought to aid in the removal of toxins and the excretion of waste products from the body.

3. Procedure and Frequency: Regular coffee enemas are recommended as part of the Gerson Therapy as part of the daily routine. The treatment includes injecting a specifically formulated coffee solution into the colon in order to facilitate detoxification and improve general health.

Other Detoxification Methods

1. Gerson Therapy stresses the need to have a healthy colon. To eliminate accumulated waste and toxins from the digestive system, colon cleaning procedures such as colonics or certain dietary habits may be advised.

2. Hydrotherapy: In Gerson Therapy, water-based therapies such as hot and cold compresses are utilized to promote the body's detoxification processes. Hydrotherapy is said to improve circulation and facilitate toxin removal via the skin.

3. Sauna treatment: Sauna treatment induces sweating, which is useful for removing toxins from the skin. Sauna treatments may be used in Gerson Therapy to boost the body's natural detoxifying systems.

To summarize, detoxification is a key component of Gerson Therapy, to improve the body's capacity to expel toxins and promote healing. Focusing on liver cleansing, using coffee enemas, and incorporating other detoxification procedures provide a complete strategy for supporting the body's natural healing processes in the context of chronic conditions.

CHAPTER FIVE

Nutritional Supplements In Gerson Therapy

Dr. Max Gerson established Gerson Therapy in the early twentieth century as a holistic and natural method to cure numerous chronic conditions, including cancer.

The emphasis on nutrition, especially via a plant-based diet, is central to this treatment. The fifth chapter dives into the vital function of nutritional supplements in Gerson Therapy, highlighting their importance in assisting the body's healing processes.

The Role Of Supplements In Supporting Healing

1. Cellular Repair: Nutritional supplements are important in enhancing the body's capacity to repair and regenerate cells. They give critical elements that typical diets may lack, assisting in the healing process.

2. Support for Detoxification: Gerson Therapy stresses detoxification as an important element of treatment. Certain nutrients aid in the detox process by boosting liver function, facilitating toxin clearance, and aiding in general body cleaning.

3. Immune System Support: A strong immune system is critical for fighting sickness and boosting general health. The supplements used in the Gerson Therapy are carefully chosen to boost immune function and provide the body with the resources it needs to combat illness.

4. Critical Organ Support: Many supplements are selected for their specialized advantages to critical organs including the liver, kidneys, and heart. Strengthening these organs is critical to the therapy's overall effectiveness.

Essential Nutrients And Their Sources

1. Vitamins: Gerson Therapy puts a high value on vitamins, believing that they are necessary for healing. Vitamin C, B-complex vitamins, and other micronutrients important for cellular function and immunological support are often included in supplements.

2. **Minerals:** Minerals such as potassium, iodine, and magnesium are essential for many physiological functions. Supplements are carefully selected to ensure that the body obtains an ideal mix of minerals for healing and health maintenance.

3. **Enzymes:** Enzymes are important for digestion and nutrition absorption. Enzyme supplementation aids the body's breakdown and assimilation of nutrients, enhancing the overall efficiency of the Gerson Therapy.

4. .Fatty acids, such as omega-3. and omega-6, are essential for cellular function and inflammation regulation. Gerson Therapy utilizes fatty acid supplementation to maintain a balanced and healthy internal environment.

Balancing The Gerson Diet With Supplements

1. Individualized Approaches: Gerson Therapy acknowledges the individuality of each person's health situation. The use of supplements is adjusted to the patient's unique requirements, enabling a personalized and successful healing process.

2. Monitoring Nutrient Intake: Regular nutrient level evaluations assist in altering supplement doses to match the body's changing demands. This diligent monitoring ensures that patients obtain the proper nutritional balance throughout their recovery process.

3. Avoiding Nutrient Excess: While supplements are necessary, it is critical to maintain a balance. Excessive consumption of some nutrients might be harmful. The Gerson Therapy method entails careful control to avoid nutritional imbalances.

Finally, Chapter Five emphasizes the critical significance of nutritional supplements in Gerson Therapy.

Individuals may better grasp the entire and holistic character of this treatment approach by understanding the role of supplements in promoting cellular repair, detoxification, immune system function, and organ health. The Gerson Therapy's effectiveness in promoting healing and general well-being is greatly enhanced by the careful selection and tailored administration of supplements.

CHAPTER SIX

Case Studies And Success Stories

In Chapter Six of our Gerson Therapy investigation, we dig into the real-life stories of people who have embraced this alternative method of healing.

These case studies and success stories, which detail instances of recovery from diverse health issues, give essential insights into the efficacy of Gerson Therapy.

Furthermore, we investigate the hurdles that people have while practicing Gerson Therapy and the techniques used to overcome these barriers.

1. Cases of Cancer Remission: Gerson Therapy has attracted attention for its involvement in cancer therapy. Numerous case studies demonstrate people who have recovered from different forms of cancer after having Gerson Therapy. These tales provide hope and motivation to individuals looking for alternative cancer therapies.

2. Beyond cancer, Gerson Therapy has been investigated as a therapy option for chronic illnesses such as diabetes, arthritis, and autoimmune disorders. Case studies illustrate situations where people have effectively treated and even reversed the

course of various illnesses using Gerson Therapy concepts.

3. Detoxification and general well-being: Gerson Therapy promotes detoxification and general well-being in addition to illness therapy. Case studies show how people who have used Gerson Therapy have experienced increased energy levels, mental clarity, and general vitality.

Documented Cases Of Healing

1. Scientific Validation: This section dives into recorded situations where Gerson Therapy has been subjected to scientific investigation, in addition to anecdotal evidence. Peer-reviewed research and medical reports add to the expanding amount of data proving Gerson Therapy's effectiveness in particular circumstances.

2. Long-term Follow-ups: Examining the long-term results of Gerson Therapy patients gives a thorough picture of its sustainability and long-term influence. We can estimate the persistence of therapy benefits by studying instances with long follow-up periods.

Overcoming Challenges In Implementation

1. Compliance with Nutrition: Gerson Therapy necessitates careful devotion to a plant-based, organic diet. Maintaining dietary compliance is one of the issues that people confront.

Personalized meal planning, nutritional counseling, and support groups may be used to overcome this difficulty.

2. **.Juicing and Treatment Routines:** The treatment requires regular juicing of fruits and vegetables, which may be time-consuming and logistically difficult. This section looks at how people have effectively included juicing into their everyday routines while overcoming practical obstacles and time restrictions.

3. **.Psychosocial and emotional support:** It is impossible to overestimate the psychological and emotional components of living with a chronic disease and sticking to a hard therapeutic regimen. Success stories emphasize the need for

psychological assistance in overcoming emotional issues, such as therapy, peer networks, and family participation.

The remarkable accounts of people who have received Gerson Therapy are highlighted in Chapter Six, demonstrating its potential for healing and recovery. This chapter is a great resource for both practitioners and persons contemplating or presently receiving Gerson Therapy since it combines real-life experiences, recorded cases, and insights for overcoming implementation obstacles.

CHAPTER SEVEN

Integrating Gerson Therapy With Conventional Medicine

Gerson Therapy And Its Relationship With Conventional Treatments

Dr. Max Gerson established Gerson Therapy in the 1920s as a comprehensive approach to treating numerous chronic illnesses, including cancer. It stresses the need for cleansing, nutritional support, and restoring the body's inherent healing power. While Gerson Therapy is regarded as an alternative or supplementary therapy, it is critical to investigate how it might be incorporated with conventional medicine to provide a complete and patient-centered treatment plan.

1.   .**Nutritional Focus:** Gerson Therapy emphasizes a plant-based diet, organic juices, and coffee enemas. Working with healthcare providers to ensure patients obtain appropriate nutrients while receiving regular treatments such as chemotherapy or radiation is part of integrating this nutritional approach with conventional medicine. Nutritional supplementation may help to reduce the negative effects of these medications and improve overall health.

2.   .**Detoxification and mainstream Treatments:** Gerson Therapy's detoxification component accords with mainstream

medicine's acknowledgment of the need of removing toxins from the body. Collaboration may concentrate on boosting the body's detoxification mechanisms, possibly improving the efficacy of traditional therapies. This may include combining Gerson Therapy procedures with traditional detox regimens.

3. .Gerson Therapy incorporates a variety of supporting therapies such as vitamins, healthy meals, and specific juices. Integrating these treatments into standard treatment protocols necessitates open communication between Gerson practitioners and traditional healthcare specialists.

Coordinated efforts may guarantee that the patient gets complete therapy without jeopardizing each approach's effectiveness.

1.   .Establishing multidisciplinary care teams comprised of Gerson therapists, oncologists, dietitians, and other healthcare experts encourages a collaborative atmosphere. This enables the sharing of information and experience, resulting in a more integrated and tailored approach to patient care.

2.   **.Patient-Centered Care:** A patient-centered approach entails adapting treatment plans to the patient's specific requirements and

preferences. Patients may benefit from a more holistic and tailored recovery path by adopting components of Gerson Therapy with conventional therapies. This integration requires shared decision-making between the patient and the healthcare team.

3.   .**Protocol Monitoring and Adjustment:** Patients having integrated therapy must be monitored regularly. This entails evaluating the patient's reaction to both Gerson Therapy and conventional therapies and making any modifications. Continuous communication between healthcare practitioners ensures that any changes are implemented in the patient's best interests.

1. **.Scientific Evidence and Research:** Gerson Therapy's scientific foundation is often questioned by critics. Collaborative efforts may include comprehensive research studies to assess the effectiveness and safety of combining Gerson Therapy with conventional therapies. This evidence-based strategy addresses skepticism while also laying a stronger platform for the combination of these two methods.

2. **.Communication and Transparency:** Addressing problems requires open and transparent communication between Gerson therapists and conventional healthcare practitioners. Sharing information regarding treatment goals,

progress, and any observable impacts (good or negative) fosters confidence and ensures that all parties are up to date on the patient's care.

3. .**Patient Education:** It is critical to educate patients about the integrated approach to create trust and comprehension. Giving patients information about the advantages, possible hazards, and projected results of combining Gerson Therapy with conventional therapies allows them to make educated health choices.

To summarize, integrating Gerson Therapy with conventional treatment necessitates a collaborative and patient-centered approach. Healthcare practitioners may collaborate to offer comprehensive treatment that maximizes the possibility of recovery by recognizing the strengths of each method and addressing issues via evidence-based procedures.

CHAPTER EIGHT

Gerson Therapy And Chronic Illnesses

Gerson Therapy In Cancer Treatment

Gerson Therapy, created by Dr. Max Gerson in the early twentieth century, rose to prominence chiefly for its use in cancer therapy. Gerson Therapy is founded on the premise that a whole-body approach that includes dietary adjustments, detoxification, and nutritional support will help the body repair itself.

1. Gerson Therapy promotes a plant-based diet that includes raw juices made from organic fruits and vegetables.

Specific nutritional supplements are also included in the regimen to help strengthen the immune system and assist in the detoxification process. Fresh, organic food is prioritized to provide important nutrients and enzymes that promote the body's natural healing capabilities.

2.   .Detoxification: Detoxification is essential in Gerson Therapy. Coffee enemas are a unique element of this regimen, designed to stimulate the liver and improve toxin clearance. The liver, a critical organ in detoxification, is thought to be crucial in the body's capacity to fight cancer.

3. PH Levels: Gerson Therapy stresses the need to maintain an alkaline environment

in the body. The suggested diet's alkaline composition is supposed to produce an unfavorable environment for cancer cells to grow. The treatment seeks to help the body's healing processes by creating an alkaline pH.

4.   .**Immune System Support:** The treatment includes immune-boosting components including vitamin and mineral supplements, which are thought to improve the immune system's capacity to identify and remove aberrant cells, including cancer cells.

Application In Other Chronic Conditions

While Gerson Therapy sprang to fame as a cancer therapy, proponents say that its principles may be applied to a variety of chronic conditions other than cancer. Gerson Therapy has been studied for a variety of chronic illnesses, including:

1. **.Autoimmune Diseases:** The Gerson diet's anti-inflammatory characteristics and focus on immune system support may be useful in controlling some autoimmune illnesses. More study is required, however, to determine its usefulness in particular autoimmune disorders.

2. **.Cardiovascular Diseases:** The Gerson diet's plant-based, low-sodium composition may be advantageous in regulating some elements of cardiovascular health. However, its efficacy as a stand-alone

treatment for cardiovascular disorders is unknown.

3. .**Digestive issues:** Gerson Therapy's focus on whole, organic meals, as well as its capacity to lower inflammation, may have consequences for those suffering from digestive issues. Again, research in this field is sparse, and individual responses to treatment may differ.

Managing Chronic Diseases With A Holistic Approach

Gerson Therapy is a comprehensive approach to treatment that emphasizes the interdependence of many biological systems as well as the significance of correcting underlying imbalances. Among the holistic principles are:

1. **Nutritional Healing:** Gerson Therapy is based on a nutrient-dense, plant-based diet that strives to provide the body with needed vitamins, minerals, and enzymes for optimum functioning.

2. **Detoxification:** In Gerson Therapy, detoxification is seen as an essential component of health maintenance. The treatment tries to eliminate accumulated toxins that may contribute to chronic diseases by boosting the body's natural detox processes.

3. Gerson Therapy acknowledges the impact of mental and emotional well-

being on physical health. The holistic approach considers stress reduction measures, positive thinking, and emotional support to be essential components.

4. Individualized therapy: Gerson Therapy stresses the necessity of personalizing therapy to the requirements of the individual. This involves taking into account the precise kind and stage of the chronic disease, as well as each patient's unique features.

While Gerson Therapy has shown promise in certain situations, it is important to highlight that its usefulness is still being debated in the medical world. Critics claim that the scientific evidence is inadequate, and that more rigorous study is required to show its efficacy across a larger range of chronic conditions. Individuals contemplating Gerson's treatment, like with any alternative treatment, should contact healthcare specialists to make educated judgments regarding its appropriateness for their unique health issues.

CHAPTER NINE

Practical Tips For Implementing Gerson Therapy

Gerson Therapy is a comprehensive method of treating and regenerating the body that includes a specialized diet, cleansing, and nutritional supplements. Implementing Gerson Therapy requires commitment, discipline, and meticulous preparation. In this chapter, we'll look at how to properly incorporate Gerson Therapy into your everyday life. We'll concentrate on building a Gerson-friendly atmosphere at home, successful food planning and preparation, and overcoming typical roadblocks along the way.

Creating A Gerson-Friendly Environment At Home

1. **.Availability of Organic Produce:** Maintain a steady supply of fresh, organic fruits and vegetables. Local organic stores, farmers' markets, and even home gardening might be great places to start. Obtaining pesticide-free, nutrient-dense vegetables should be prioritized.

2. **.Juicing Station:** Set aside a section of your kitchen for juicing. For effective and easy juicing, invest in a high-quality juicer, cutting boards, and sharp knives.

To speed up the process, keep the area clean and orderly.

3. .Storage and refrigeration are critical for big quantities of fresh food. Consider purchasing a refrigerator with plenty of storage capacity for fruits and vegetables. Organize the fridge properly to minimize spoiling and guarantee simple access.

4. .**Water Filtration:** Gerson Therapy stresses the need to drink clean, uncontaminated water. Purchase a dependable water filtration system to guarantee that the water used in treatment is free of pollutants and contaminants.

5. .**Natural Cleaning Products:** To keep your living area clean, use natural and non-

toxic cleaning products. This is necessary to prevent exposure to potentially toxic compounds that might impede the detoxification process.

Meal Planning And Preparation

1. .**Weekly Meal Plans:** Set aside time each week to construct a comprehensive meal plan. Plan your meals ahead of time, taking into account the necessary juices, plant-based meals, and supplements. Maintaining consistency is easier with a set approach.

2. .**Batch cooking:** Make the cooking process more efficient by preparing bigger quantities of particular dishes. This may save time over the week while also

ensuring that Gerson-approved meals are easily accessible.

3.   .**Preparation of items:** Wash, chop, and prepare items ahead of time to speed up dinner preparation. Having pre-prepared veggies and fruits might help you stick to the program, particularly on hectic days.

4.   .**Variety and Creativity:** Experiment with various recipes and variants to keep meals interesting. Experimenting with herbs and spices may add taste without jeopardizing the diet's curative properties.

Overcoming Common Obstacles

1.   .**Social Difficulties:** Discuss the food limitations of Gerson Therapy freely with friends and family.

Plan ahead of time for social occasions, and bring your own Gerson-friendly foods to offer.

2. **.Time Management:** Gerson Therapy requires a substantial time commitment, particularly during juicing. To handle stress, create a regimen that meets the demands of treatment and emphasizes self-care.

3. **.Financial Considerations:** While organic vegetables and supplements might be expensive, explore less expensive alternatives. To save money, look into local markets, bulk purchasing, and seasonal vegetables. To relieve financial stress, plan and budget for the treatment.

4.   .Engage in an emotional support network, whether it's friends, family, or online groups. Maintaining motivation and handling the hurdles that may come throughout the Gerson Therapy journey need emotional support.

Finally, applying Gerson Therapy requires a proactive and systematic approach. Creating a Gerson-friendly atmosphere, rigorous meal preparation, and addressing typical hurdles can all help you integrate Gerson Therapy into your everyday life more smoothly and successfully. Keep in mind that consistency and determination are essential for obtaining the full advantages of this holistic treatment strategy.

CHAPTER TEN

The Future Of Gerson Therapy

Gerson Therapy, which was created by Dr. Max Gerson in the early twentieth century, has been the focus of continuous study and development, to improve its efficacy and expand its accessibility.

We investigate the newest breakthroughs in Gerson Therapy, possible protocols inspired by Gerson's concepts, and initiatives to increase knowledge and accessibility.

1.   .Ongoing study is being conducted to investigate the scientific validity of Gerson Therapy. Clinical trials and research are required to offer solid data supporting the effectiveness of treatment in treating different illnesses, including cancer. Researchers are looking at how Gerson Therapy affects the immune system, inflammation, and cellular health.

2.   **.Nutritional Optimization:** Scientists are working to improve the nutritional components of Gerson Therapy. This entails discovering particular nutrients, antioxidants, and bioactive chemicals that are critical to the efficacy of the treatment.

The objective is to fine-tune the dietary factors to maximize therapeutic results.

3.   .Future advancements may involve a customized medicine approach, customizing Gerson-inspired procedures to particular patient profiles. Advances in genetic and molecular studies may aid in the identification of particular food and lifestyle changes that can maximize treatment for each patient.

Potential Advancements In Gerson-Inspired Protocols

1.   .**Integration with Modern Medicine:** A potential area of investigation is collaboration between Gerson Therapy and conventional medical therapies.

Combining Gerson Therapy's holistic approach with focused medical therapies may improve overall patient results, resulting in a complete and integrated approach to healthcare.

2.   **.Detoxification Protocol Innovations:** Research in Gerson Therapy is centered on improving and creating detoxification regimens. Future Gerson-inspired regimens may include advanced strategies for supporting the liver, improving lymphatic drainage, and maximizing cellular detoxification.

3.   **.Technological Integration:** The use of technology, like as wearable gadgets and health monitoring applications, may help people adhere to Gerson-inspired practices

more easily. Healthcare practitioners may give more tailored and effective counsel if they have real-time data on eating habits, physical activity, and biomarkers.

Promoting Awareness And Accessibility

1. .**Education Initiatives:** It is critical to raise knowledge about Gerson Therapy via educational efforts. Public lectures, internet materials, and cooperation with healthcare institutions may help debunk myths about the treatment and promote informed decision-making.

2. .**Patient Support Networks:** Creating support networks for Gerson Therapy patients may help them stick to their treatment and

get better results. Online forums, local support groups, and patient advocacy organizations may all provide a place for people to share their stories, suggestions, and emotional support.

3.   .**Training Treatment Professionals:** To integrate Gerson Therapy into mainstream treatment, healthcare professionals must be trained in its concepts and practice. Continuing education seminars and workshops may equip healthcare personnel to give knowledgeable counsel and assistance to Gerson Therapy patients.

4.   .**Research financing:** Obtaining financing for Gerson Therapy research is critical for expanding its legitimacy and acceptability

in the medical world. Collaboration with academic institutes, government organizations, and private foundations may offer the resources needed for serious scientific study.

To summarize, the future of Gerson Therapy is bright, thanks to continuing research, prospective protocol changes, and attempts to raise knowledge and accessibility. As the therapeutic landscape advances, incorporating Gerson-inspired treatments into mainstream healthcare procedures will need a thorough and collaborative strategy.

Dr. Max Gerson invented Gerson Therapy in the early twentieth century, and it remains a contentious but interesting alternative method to treating different maladies, most notably cancer. It is based on the idea that a well-balanced diet, cleansing, and supplements may help the body's natural healing capabilities.

While the treatment has anecdotal success stories and ardent supporters, its effectiveness has yet to be scientifically validated by large-scale, controlled clinical research. Critics point out the lack of clear data to back up its promises and warn against forsaking traditional therapies in favor of Gerson Therapy.

Its focus on nutrient-dense diets, cleansing, and general lifestyle adjustments, on the other hand, is sound. The emphasis on fresh organic fruits, vegetables, and juices is consistent with long-standing health recommendations for a well-balanced diet. The therapy's emphasis on avoiding processed foods, coffee, and alcohol encourages a better lifestyle as well.

However, the strict dietary regimen, intensive juicing, and coffee enemas involved in Gerson Therapy may make adherence difficult for many people. Furthermore, relying solely on natural remedies and avoiding conventional medicine may pose risks for certain conditions that necessitate immediate and specific medical interventions.

To summarize, while Gerson Therapy provides a holistic approach to health and healing, its scientific validity and universal applicability are still debated. Individuals considering alternative treatments must engage in informed discussions with healthcare providers, weigh potential benefits against risks, and make decisions that are consistent with their overall health needs and beliefs. While incorporating aspects of Gerson Therapy, such as a plant-based diet and lifestyle changes, into a broader health regimen may provide some benefits, its complete replacement for conventional medical treatments should be approached with caution and professional guidance.

THE END

www.ingramcontent.com/pod-product-compliance
Lightning Source LLC
Chambersburg PA
CBHW050738260726
48661CB00001B/291